Couple's evening

Creation and illustration
LOVE AND MORE EDITION

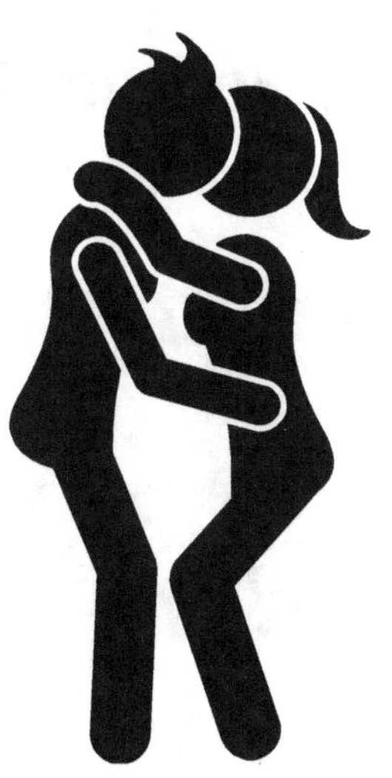

INTRODUCTION

This game is for couples who want to get to know each other better or for those who want to (re)discover each other and promote more harmonious relationships, in a playful, innovative and sensual way.

....

Playing together brings joy and greater resilience to your relationship. It can also heal any resentments and disagreements you have. Through play, we learn to trust each other and feel safe

"The search for pleasure for two is to make the other want to do it again".

ADVICE

Before sex:

- Brush your teeth to remove odors from your mouth. Also, try not to eat unpleasant foods before sex, such as onions and garlic.

- Make sure you smell good - the freshest smell is after a shower and the worst smell is sweat! Women in particular are sensitive to smell.

- Add small personal touches to your environment to create the right atmosphere: your favorite playlist, dimmed lights, scented candles, anything that can help enhance the moments to come,

- Kisses, caresses and other sweet words reinforce the complicity and create a delicious harmony between the partners... So don't send them in a few minutes!

"Intimate hygiene is associated with body cleanliness, self-respect and respect for one's partner"

EXPLANATION OF THE GAME

The rules of the game are simple:

Place yourselves in front of each other, each in turn ask your partner a question, every 6 questions, you will have the right to choose an action, the goal is to discover each other through the answers and exchanges related to the questions and actions (BONUS cards will sometimes be proposed)

Bonus cards will be cut out at the end of the book, place them next to you

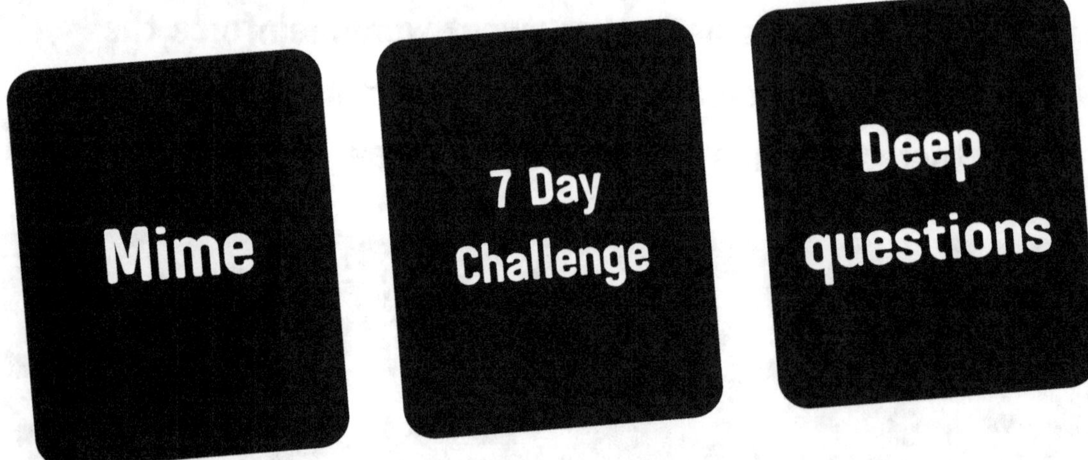

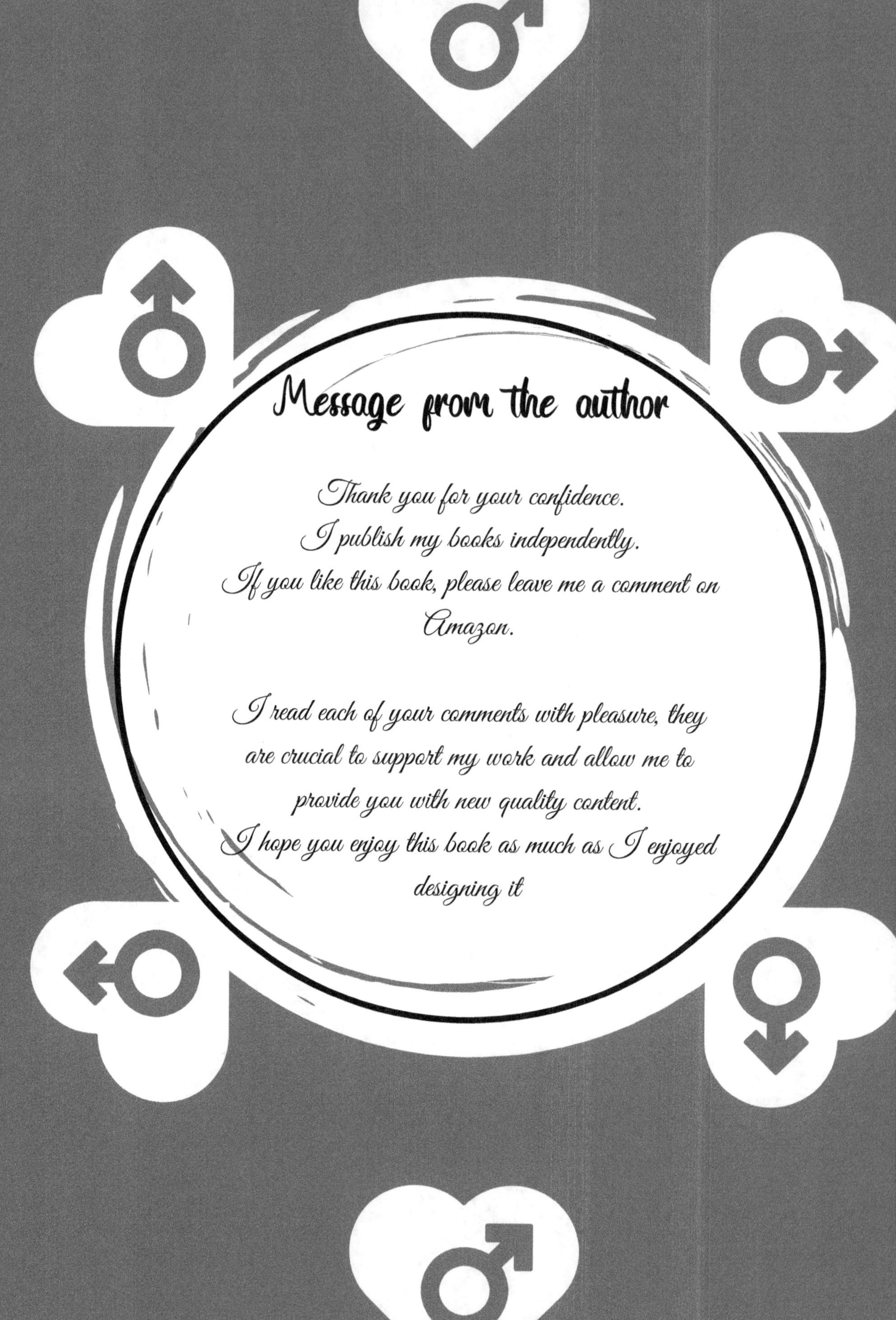

Message from the author

Thank you for your confidence.
I publish my books independently.
If you like this book, please leave me a comment on Amazon.

I read each of your comments with pleasure, they are crucial to support my work and allow me to provide you with new quality content.
I hope you enjoy this book as much as I enjoyed designing it

1

What does a perfect evening for two look like?

2

The 3 values you absolutely want to pass on to your children?

3

If you were convinced I was making a bad decision, what would you do?

4

What language would you like to learn?

5

What is your biggest fantasy?

6

Which part of my body do you prefer?

ACTION 1

Gently approach your partner without telling her the action and kiss her neck sensually for about 30 seconds?

OU

ACTION 2

Look your other half in the eyes, in silence and kiss her on the mouth with a lot of passion

7

What sport would you like to try that you have never done before?

8

What is your definition of the word romantic?

9

Your biggest complex?

10

Who is the person you admire the most? Why ?

11

What is your definition of the word responsible?

12

What makes you fall for me?

ACTION 3

Stand behind your partner and start massaging his or her shoulders and back with maximum delicacy and softness for 3 minutes without saying a word

OU

ACTION 4

Lick the earlobes of your other half with amazing sensuality for 30 seconds

BONUS cards

Make Rock, Paper, Scissors up to 3

The winner chooses the theme of the card for his or her other half, who must either answer the question asked or perform the action requested

Mime

7 Day Challenge

Deep questions

13

Name 3 qualities and 3 defects that characterize you!

14

How many children would you like to have?

15

What is your biggest fear in a relationship?

16

What is the nicest surprise I could give you?

17

What is your ideal romantic weekend?

18

What's the dumbest thing you've ever done?

ACTION 5

Without saying the action, ask your half to put a blindfold on his head, ask him to lie down, you are now going to caress his whole body (on the clothes), insist well on the buttocks and the chest, the whole gently and very slowly during 5 minutes

OU

ACTION 6

Ask your partner to take off your top and then ask her to kiss your chest for at least 1 minute

19

What generally attracts you to a man/woman?

20

What are your favorite kinds of movies?

21

What is your favorite food?

22

If you had to live in another country, which one would it be? Why ?

23

What is the most important character trait for you?

24

What's the worst thing you've ever eaten?

ACTION 7

Turn off the lights or close the blinds and get into complete darkness.

Stand up, hug your partner and rub against each other's private parts, kissing warmly for 3 minutes

OU

ACTION 8

Ask your partner to take off the top of your clothes and then ask her to kiss your chest for at least 1 minute

BONUS cards

Make Rock, Paper, Scissors up to 3

The winner chooses the theme of the card for his or her other half, who must either answer the question asked or perform the action requested

Mime

7 Day Challenge

Deep questions

25

What nickname would you like me
to call you?

26

Do you prefer to do it in the dark or
with a little light?

27

Do you like reading?
If so, what is your favorite book?

28

What name would you give if we had a boy?

29

Are you more sea or mountain?

30

What part of your body do you complex?

ACTION 9

Undress each other gently and stay in your underwear only

OU

ACTION 10

Do Pierre Feuille Ciseau, the first to arrive at 3 selected points who undresses (in underwear)

31

What is your favorite movie?

32

Would you like to have a pet? If so, which one?

33

What is your biggest regret?

34

What is the flaw you hate
most about me?

35

What are the qualities you like best
about me?

36

If we were locked in an elevator for
3 hours, what would we do?

ACTION 11

Get into the missionary position and rub yourself gently for 2 minutes

OU

ACTION 12

The lady lies on her stomach and the man rubs himself against her for 2 minutes

BONUS cards

Make Rock, Paper, Scissors up to 3

The winner chooses the theme of the card for his or her other half, who must either answer the question asked or perform the action requested

Mime

7 Day Challenge

Deep questions

37

What is your favorite activity to do with me?

38

What would be the craziest thing you would be willing to do for me?

39

5 small everyday things that make you happy?

40

What attracts you most to me?

41

What are the qualities you like best about me?

42

Should a love relationship be passionate, wild, routine?

ACTION 13

Kiss languidly the chest of your other half for 2 minutes

OU

ACTION 14

Stroke your partner's buttocks for 1 minute

43

What is the greatest strength of our couple?

44

How long did it take you to realize that you were in love?

45

Professionally, where do you see yourself in 3 years?

46

What is the sexiest thing about me?

47

What do you think is my worst flaw?

48

Describe me one sentence

Take off each other's underwear

BONUS cards

Make Rock, Paper, Scissors up to 3

The winner chooses the theme of the card for his or her other half, who must either answer the question asked or perform the action requested

Mime	7 Day Challenge	Deep questions

49

A naughty scenario that turns you on?

50

What do you think is my worst flaw?

51

What is the best day of your life?

52

If you could change one part of your body, which would you choose?

53

For you, what is love?

54

Who is the more stubborn of the two?

ACTION 16
Masturbate your partner for 1 minute

OU

ACTION 17
Mister stimulates the clitoris of Madam during 1 minute

55

Which sexy costume would you like me to wear?

56

What is your favorite song?

57

What is your favorite restaurant?

58

Have you ever looked at my cell phone?

59

Do you prefer dogs or cats?

60

What is your favorite quote?

ACTION 18

Missionary position: Mister rubs his penis against the clitoris of Madam during 2 minutes (without penetration)

OU

ACTION 19

Mister is lying on his back: Madam climbs on him and rubs herself against his penis for 2 minutes

BONUS cards

The winner chooses the theme of the card for his or her other half, who must either answer the question asked or perform the action requested

Mime	7 Day Challenge	Deep questions

61

What is the scariest thing that has ever happened to you?

62

What is your best memory?

63

Do you prefer a dominant, submissive or neutral partner? Why ?

64

Who is your biggest confidant?

65

What do you like most about me?

66

What is the greatest strength of our couple?

The lady has her hands tied and her eyes blindfolded, while the man does what he wants with her for 5 minutes without using his hands (without penetration)

OU

Mister has his hands tied and his eyes blindfolded, while Madam does what she wants with him for 5 minutes (without penetration)

BONUS cards

Make Rock, Paper, Scissors up to 3

The winner chooses the theme of the card for his or her other half, who must either answer the question asked or perform the action requested

| Mime | 7 Day Challenge | Deep questions |

and now...

The pleasure

is all yours!

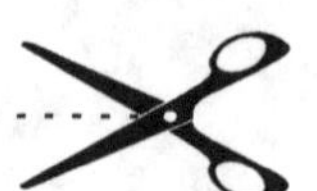

Mime

Mime

Mime

Mime

Mime

Mime

Cutting cards 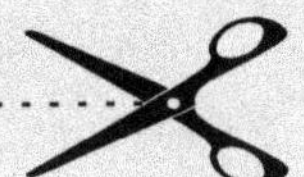

Mimics a person defrauding the gates of the Parisian metro

Mimics a fireman saving a child from a fire

Mimic a Komodo dragon wandering in the Thai bushes

Mimic your reaction to a condom cracking during sex

Mimics a drunk guy hitting on a nightclub

Mime a one-legged unicorn

Cutting cards 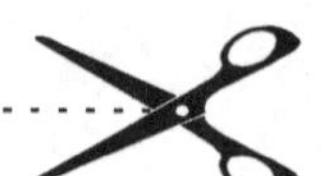

7 Day Challenge

7 Day Challenge

7 Day Challenge

7 Day Challenge

7 Day Challenge

7 Day Challenge

Cutting cards

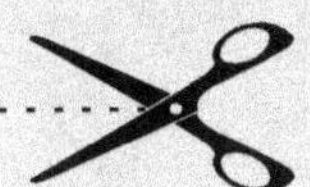

Create a photo album of the two of you and have it printed at low cost on the internet

Buy this book on Amazon and send it to a couple of friends to give them a wonderful surprise

Buy your partner an original and nice gift for less than 5€.

Prepare a candlelight dinner by cooking yourself or have an original meal delivered

Have sex in your car in the middle of the day in a place where there is no one

Fait un massage de 30 minutes à ta moitié à l'aide huile

Cutting cards

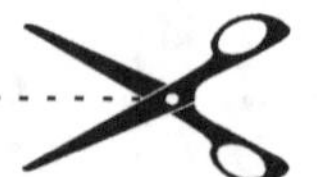

Deep questions

Deep questions

Deep questions

Deep questions

Deep questions

Deep questions

Cartes à découper

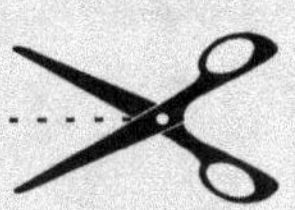

Take 5 minutes and tell your life story to your other half, with as much detail as possible

Is there something you've been dreaming of doing for a long time? Why haven't you done it?

Do you think your childhood was happier than most people's?

Share a personal problem and ask your significant other how they would handle it

Complete this sentence: "I wish I had someone to share..." and explain why

What subject is too serious to laugh about? and what does your other half think?

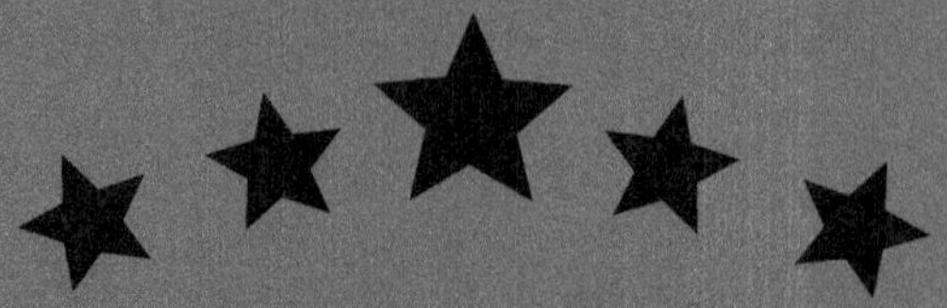

THANK YOU FOR PURCHASING OUR BOOK!

If you like this book, we would appreciate your review on Amazon.

To do so, go to the Amazon page of this book and click on "Write my review".

THANK YOU VERY MUCH!

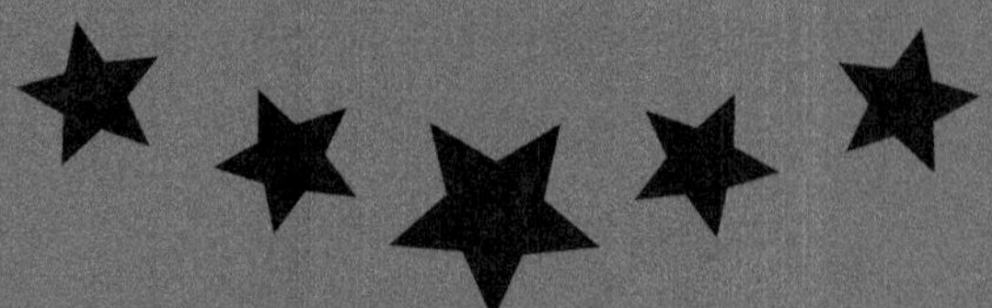